THE MEDICINE-FREE,

ILLNESS-FREE SERIES

WHY NATURAL HEALTH IS THE FUTURE

Millions Are Optimizing

Their Health Naturally

Forest Yin, DAOM, L.Ac.

First Edition: May 2025

Published by Ashi Healing

www.AshiHealing.com

Paperback ISBN: 978-1-967735-00-6

eBook ISBN: 978-1-967735-01-3

Printed in the United States of America

Medical Disclaimer:

This book is for informational purposes only and is not intended as medical advice. The author and publisher assume no responsibility for how the information is used. Readers should consult a healthcare professional before making any health-related decisions.

Forward

Nature is the origin of life, the origin of healing, and remains a guiding force in human well-being. Long before modern science developed medicine in laboratories, nature provided everything the human body needed to survive, and to sustain life. The food we eat, the herbs we gather, the minerals beneath our feet, and the sun above us are all part of an intelligent and interconnected system that has long nourished and supported the human body.

This truth has been known across cultures for thousands of years, and it is echoed in sacred texts. In the Book of Genesis, the Garden of Eden was described as a paradise where "every tree that is pleasant to the sight and good for food" was made available to humankind (Genesis 2:9). Some scholars believe this refers not only to nourishment, but also to the ability to contribute to human well-being. It becomes even more clear in Ezekiel 47:12: "The fruit thereof shall be for meat, and the leaf thereof for medicine."

Somewhere along the way, modern culture drifted from this wisdom. Many now believe that healing must come through synthetic drugs, surgeries, or man-made interventions, forgetting that the foundation of human health has always been rooted in nature. But what if well-being isn't only about medical breakthroughs, but also about reconnecting with what has always been available to us?

What if the body doesn't need to be forced to function differently, but simply supported, nourished, balanced, and reminded of what it already knows? What if illness is not the enemy, but a signal that we've fallen out of balance, and out of sync with nature?

This is not to dismiss the value of conventional medicine. We are deeply grateful for its life-saving capabilities in emergencies and acute care. But when it comes to supporting long-term vitality and encouraging balance, it may be time to return to the source.

In addition to thousands of years of lived wisdom, modern science is now exploring the potential of many natural approaches. What was once viewed as "alternative" is now increasingly recognized as part of a broader wellness conversation.

This book, and the entire *Medicine-Free, Illness-Free Series*, is rooted in this truth: Nature not only gave us life. Many believe it holds the power to support our well-being. And many of these natural approaches are now being studied and better understood through science.

Healing is not something we must force or fear. It is something we can encourage, by gently supporting the body, naturally.

Dr. Forest Yin, DAOM, L.Ac.

Author, *The Medicine-Free, Illness-Free Series*

Founder, Ashi Healing and Acupuncture Inc.

Important Disclaimer

The supplements, therapies, and natural approaches discussed in *The Medicine-Free, Illness-Free Series* are intended to support general wellness and the body's natural balance. They are not intended to diagnose, treat, cure, or prevent any disease and have not been evaluated by the U.S. Food and Drug Administration (FDA).

These books are provided for educational purposes only and are not a substitute for professional medical advice, diagnosis, or treatment. Always consult your physician or a licensed healthcare provider before starting any new supplement, therapy, or wellness routine, especially if you are pregnant, nursing, have a medical condition, or are taking medications.

The content in this series is informed by two sources: summaries of available scientific research, presented as "Science-Informed Solution Benefits", and aggregated user feedback, presented as "Customer-Reported Solution Benefits". These are intended to inform and inspire, but they reflect general patterns, not guarantees. Individual results will vary.

The phrase *"Medicine-Free, Illness-Free"* reflects a natural wellness philosophy and is not a medical claim or promise of outcome.

By reading this book, you agree to take full responsibility for your personal health choices and to seek guidance from qualified health professionals when needed.

Contents

Preface

Do you face health challenges that seem insurmountable? Perhaps you experience ongoing discomfort or any kind of imbalance that disrupts your daily life. Do you struggle to sleep, facing restless nights more often than you'd like? Do you find it difficult to feel steady and supported in your overall health and energy? Are you navigating ongoing wellness concerns or looking for natural ways to support your long-term well-being?

Do digestive issues like bloating, occasional reflux, or general stomach discomfort affect your day? Do you feel drained, fatigued, or lacking energy and strength? Are you experiencing brain fog or difficulty focusing? Do you sometimes feel emotionally low or overwhelmed? Or perhaps it's something else, physical or mental, that constantly disrupts your sense of well-being.

Have you explored conventional options but found yourself still searching for something that felt right for your body? Have you tried supplements but felt unsure where to start? and found it hard to know what truly supported your needs?

Are you searching for simple, natural health options that are easy to use and sustain, without the discomfort that sometimes comes with other choices? Options that may help you feel more balanced in the present and gently support your long-term wellness?

If you answer yes to any of these questions, then *The Medicine-Free, Illness-Free Series* is here to guide you.

The *Medicine-Free, Illness-Free Series* is designed to introduce you to all-natural, whole-food-based supplements and simple, science-informed approaches that may support your well-being. Everything in this series is rooted in nature and reflects tools that many people have found helpful for supporting their balance, comfort, and overall vitality.

The solutions in this book series are not just theoretical. They've been explored by many individuals seeking support with sleep, digestion, energy, stress, and more, as part of their efforts to feel more aligned and resilient in their lives. These aren't just remedies I've researched, and they're approaches I personally use and have seen resonate with others over time.

With *The Medicine-Free, Illness-Free Series*, you no longer have to search aimlessly for natural solutions, as many widely used nature-based options are right here to explore and consider. And it's designed to be simple, offering support in ways that easily fit into daily life. These solutions can be integrated gradually into your routine and maintained over time, as part of a wellness approach that doesn't require major lifestyle changes.

Wellness should feel natural, empowering, and sustainable. That's what this series is here to offer—tools to support your body with ease and confidence.

Why Natural Health Is the Future is the first book in *The Medicine-Free, Illness-Free Series*, created to provide a foundational understanding of natural health. While this introductory book does not offer specific therapy protocols, it will expand your awareness of how natural health approaches are being explored by many as part of their personal wellness journeys. It explores why chronic health challenges are increasing and how that has led many people to consider nature-based strategies. You'll learn how conventional medicine and natural health each play different roles, and why many are now exploring both. This book also explores how natural therapies may support well-being by helping the body maintain its natural balance. It lays the foundation for the full series, which presents simple, science-informed approaches to support wellness in daily life. While each person's journey is different, many have shared positive experiences after exploring the kinds of therapies introduced here.

Rather than making promises or claims, this series presents a structured, educational approach based on two pillars:

Science-Informed Solution Benefits: a review of what scientific research indicates about the potential of each supplement or therapy.

Customer-Reported Solution Benefits: an analysis of thousands of real-world user reviews, capturing what people say they experience most often when using each natural solution.

This combined method allows you to explore each natural option with confidence, grounded in data and real-life experience, while staying within safe and compliant boundaries.

Each of the books in this series focuses on a specific type of natural therapy. Whether it's herbs, mushrooms, amino acids, animal organ supplements, or core nutrient protocols, you'll find clear explanations, structured insights, and practical guidance that can help you discover which approaches feel most supportive for your unique needs, without requiring drastic lifestyle changes.

Our goal is simple: to empower you with trusted, science-informed, and real-world-tested knowledge. By understanding your options and how they may gently support your health, you can take meaningful steps toward balance, energy, and resilience, on your own terms.

Let's begin the journey.

Meet Dr. Forest Yin, DAOM, L.Ac.

Professionally known as Forest Yin, my official name is Jie Yin, while also known as 尹明杰 in the Chinese speaking communities.

For most of my professional life, I was known as a high-tech executive, problem-solver, and innovator in information security and technologies. In leadership roles at Oracle, Schwab, and Wells Fargo, I developed and managed advanced security solutions, ensuring stability, efficiency, and high performance in a fast-paced, high-stakes environment.

But after work, I was deeply immersed in another world, the science of natural health.

My journey into Traditional Chinese Medicine (TCM) began in college, when I first studied the *Huang Di Nei Jing (Yellow Emperor's Classic of Internal Medicine)* alongside my Physics degree. While excelling in my tech career, I continued to research, experiment, and apply natural healing principles, seeking ways to optimize health, energy, and resilience, not just for myself, but for those around me.

Recognizing the profound impact of natural medicine on long-term health and performance, I pursued formal training, becoming a Licensed Acupuncturist (L.Ac.) in 2018 and earning my Doctorate in Acupuncture and Oriental Medicine (DAOM) in 2019. Since then,

I have supported individuals around the world in improving their vitality, resilience, and sense of well-being through natural methods. This led me to found Ashi Healing and Acupuncture Inc. and become a Professor and Doctoral Advisor at the University of East-West Medicine, where I mentor future practitioners in the art of TCM.

Applying Systems Thinking to Health & Healing

In high-tech, solving problems requires understanding systems, identifying vulnerabilities, and optimizing performance. I apply the same mindset to health. Instead of treating symptoms, I look at the root cause, like debugging a system. Instead of temporary fixes, I focus on long-term balance and resilience, like designing sustainable architecture. Instead of pharmaceutical dependency, I seek efficient, natural approaches that support function and balance gently, without the common side effects associated with conventional options, like optimizing system performance.

While many of my colleagues in the tech and finance industries thrived in their careers, I also saw the toll of chronic stress, burnout, autoimmune conditions, and lifestyle-related illnesses. Like many professionals, they pushed their limits, until their bodies pushed back. This is where natural approaches can make a difference.

A Philosophy Rooted in Balance & Natural Healing

At Ashi Healing, my approach complements conventional care by focusing on identifying underlying imbalances and supporting the body's natural self-regulation through Traditional Chinese Medicine and holistic strategies.

The name "Ashi (阿是)" comes from a fundamental concept in Chinese medicine, that moment of realization when healing feels real. In Chinese, "Ashi" means "Ahh, Yes!", the instant when your body recognizes exactly what it needs. This guiding philosophy shapes everything I do, from acupuncture to natural health solutions.

Through the precise use of Chinese Herbal Medicine and modern whole-food-based natural supplements like herbs and mushrooms, I have helped individuals support their energy and balance naturally, using simple, sustainable tools that complement or reduce the need for pharmaceutical interventions when appropriate.

My mission is simple: to help people pursue wellness and resilience, naturally and sustainably.

Integrating Ancient Wisdom with Modern Innovation

Chinese Herbal Medicine has been refined for thousands of years. But today, we can take it further, combining ancient wisdom with modern research and a strategic, data-driven approach to health optimization.

At Ashi Healing, I personalize each protocol based on the individual's needs, whether it's boosting energy, reducing stress, improving cognitive function, or addressing chronic health concerns. Many of the people I work with are busy professionals seeking practical, time-efficient strategies to support their health without disrupting their demanding schedules.

Looking for More Information and Support

To learn more about my personalized approach to Chinese Herbal Therapy and whole-food-based supplements, visit AshiHealing.com. You'll find additional resources and simple ways to take the next step in your healing journey, whenever you're ready.

And remember, this book is just one part of *The Medicine-Free, Illness-Free Series*. Each volume explores a different pillar of natural healing, from herbs and mushrooms to amino acids, detoxification, and grounding, offering you a complete path to support your balance and well-being through nature-based strategies.

The Growing Challenge of Modern Health Issues

The World Health Organization (WHO) defines health as "a state of complete physical, mental, and social well-being, not merely the absence of disease or infirmity." While this definition has existed for decades, many would agree it feels more relevant today than ever before. In an era of fast-paced living, high stress, and increasing environmental burdens, achieving this level of complete well-being has become a growing challenge across the globe.

Despite incredible advancements in diagnostics, pharmaceuticals, and surgical technology, millions of people continue to struggle with persistent health concerns. Many of these challenges are not the result of rare infections or emergencies, but instead stem from long-term patterns of stress, inactivity, processed diets, disrupted sleep, and toxic exposures. Public health data continues to show rising rates of metabolic imbalance, cardiovascular strain, immune dysfunction, and emotional burnout in populations worldwide.

This has prompted an important shift. More and more individuals are no longer looking only to manage symptoms. They are beginning to ask different questions:

What is causing this imbalance? How can I support my body before a crisis occurs? Is there another way to build true resilience?

These questions are at the heart of a global movement, one that is revisiting nature's role in restoring balance and supporting vitality. From ancient herbal systems to modern nutritional science, people are turning toward integrative, supportive approaches that work with the body, rather than against it.

Widespread Chronic Wellness Challenges

Over the past several decades, chronic illness has quietly become one of the most pressing public health challenges of our time. Once considered conditions that primarily affected older adults or at-risk populations, chronic diseases are now widespread across all age groups, income levels, and regions of the world. What was once an exception is now a norm.

According to the World Health Organization (WHO), chronic diseases, also referred to as non-communicable diseases, are responsible for over 70% of all deaths globally, accounting for more than 41 million lives lost each year. In high-income countries such as the United States, this number rises even further. Chronic conditions are now the leading cause of death and disability in the United States, representing approximately 90% of all deaths annually. These include long-term health conditions that persist for years and often require ongoing care and management, placing a substantial burden not only on individuals and families but also on healthcare systems and national economies.

The number of people living with chronic health conditions continues to grow year after year. Globally, the affected population has risen from approximately 1.2 billion in 2010 to an estimated 1.66 billion by 2023, an increase of nearly 38%. In the United States alone, the number of individuals diagnosed with one or more chronic illnesses rose from 125 million in 2010 to over 162 million in 2023, marking a 30% increase in just over a decade. These trends show no signs of slowing.

Perhaps even more concerning is the early onset of chronic conditions among younger populations. According to the most recent data from the Centers for Disease Control and Prevention (CDC), more than 40% of school-aged children in the United States are reported to have at least one ongoing health condition. Among adults, over 60% are living with one or more chronic diseases, and approximately 40% are managing two or more at the same time. These statistics illustrate the extent to which chronic health issues have become embedded in the daily lives of the majority of Americans.

The financial impact is equally staggering. According to the Centers for Disease Control and Prevention (CDC), 90% of the nation's $4.5

trillion in annual healthcare expenditures are for people with chronic and mental health conditions. That amounts to about $4 trillion per year spent on managing long-term conditions, many of which require frequent medical visits, ongoing prescriptions, hospital care, and long-term support. Globally, the economic burden is estimated to reach over $47 trillion by 2030 if current trends continue, according to data from the World Economic Forum. These numbers reflect not only the rising cost of care but the sheer scale of the challenge facing governments, health systems, employers, and individuals.

What is now clear is that chronic illness is not an isolated issue. It has become a dominant force shaping the modern health landscape crisis that touches nearly every household and every demographic. As the prevalence continues to grow, the weight of these conditions places enormous stress on healthcare infrastructure, economic productivity, and overall societal well-being.

Chronic illness is no longer a background concern. It is the defining health crisis of our generation.

The Impact of Lifestyle on Health

Across the globe, shifting patterns in daily life are having a profound effect on long-term health. While genetics, environment, and access to care all play a role, a growing body of public health data points to modern lifestyle as one of the most consistent factors influencing overall well-being. The way people eat, move, sleep, and respond to stress has changed dramatically in recent decades, and not always for the better.

Diet is one of the most visible areas of concern. In the United States, the typical dietary pattern has moved far from its whole-food roots. According to the Centers for Disease Control and Prevention (CDC), over 60% of the calories consumed by American adults now come from ultra-processed foods—products that are heavily refined, stripped of fiber and nutrients, and often high in added sugars, sodium, and industrial fats. These foods may offer convenience and long shelf life, but they often deliver limited nutritional value. In fact, fewer than 1 in 10 adults in the U.S. consume the recommended daily amount of vegetables, and most fall short on fiber, potassium, magnesium, and essential vitamins. Globally, the trend is similar: diets are becoming more calorie-dense but nutrient-poor, raising concern among nutrition experts and public health officials.

Alongside poor diet quality is a steep decline in physical activity. The World Health Organization reports that approximately 1.4 billion adults worldwide do not meet recommended physical activity levels. In the United States, the CDC estimates that only about 24% of adults meet the physical activity guidelines for both aerobic and muscle-strengthening activities. For children and teens, the numbers are equally troubling: only one in four high school students meets the daily activity recommendation. Sedentary behavior, defined as prolonged sitting or minimal movement, is increasingly common due to the nature of modern work, transportation, and leisure. Desk jobs, long commutes, and screen-based entertainment have collectively reduced the amount of natural movement built into daily life.

The effects of this shift extend far beyond muscle tone or physical fitness. Physical inactivity has been associated with decreased circulation, lower energy levels, cognitive dullness, and poor sleep quality. When combined with diets that lack adequate nutrients, this creates a scenario where the body may be operating in a state of depletion, even if food is abundant and the lifestyle is technologically advanced.

Sleep is another cornerstone of health that has been affected by modern habits. Studies from the National Sleep Foundation indicate that 35% of U.S. adults report sleeping fewer than seven hours per night, the minimum amount recommended for overall health. The rise of artificial light, evening screen use, and round-the-clock digital communication has disrupted circadian rhythms for millions. Sleep deprivation doesn't just cause fatigue, it can influence hormone regulation, immune function, and mood stability, creating ripple effects that impact daily performance and long-term wellness.

Stress has also emerged as a dominant force in modern life. According to the American Psychological Association's most recent "Stress in America" survey, more than 75% of adults report experiencing moderate to high stress levels in the past month. Work, finances, and health concerns top the list, and chronic stress is increasingly seen as a hidden driver of many physical and emotional challenges. Though stress itself is a natural response, extended exposure without adequate recovery can lead to ongoing tension, mental fatigue, poor sleep, and diminished vitality.

These patterns, nutritionally poor diets, physical inactivity, insufficient sleep, and unrelenting stress, do not occur in isolation. They interact, often reinforcing one another in subtle and compounding ways. Together, they form a lifestyle landscape that places unprecedented demands on the body, often without providing the restorative practices needed to maintain balance.

This convergence of lifestyle challenges is being documented across countries, age groups, and income levels. While the specifics may vary by region, the broader concern is universal: many of today's daily habits, once seen as markers of progress or convenience, are now recognized as contributing to a decline in everyday vitality and long-term health resilience. The modern lifestyle, in its current form, has introduced new obstacles to feeling well, functioning clearly, and aging gracefully.

The Impact of Environmental Issues and Diet on Health

In today's world, the connection between environment, agriculture, and nutrition is becoming harder to ignore. While lifestyle habits like movement, rest, and stress clearly shape our well-being, the environmental quality of the food we eat and the systems that produce it also play a growing role in our health outcomes.

Modern agricultural practices, industrialized food production, and widespread chemical use have fundamentally transformed the way food is grown, processed, and consumed. In many regions, the shift from traditional farming methods to large-scale industrial models has prioritized speed, volume, and shelf life over soil health and nutrient preservation. At the same time, highly processed foods, designed for convenience and taste, have become dietary staples for millions around the world.

These changes have created a nutritional paradox. While food is more abundant and accessible than ever, concerns are rising about what that food actually delivers to the human body. Many people now consume far more calories than past generations, yet may be absorbing fewer of the vitamins, minerals, and plant-based compounds the body needs for its natural functions. This disconnect is raising questions across the health community about whether modern food systems are supporting or straining long-term well-being.

In the sections that follow, we will explore three critical issues: the depletion of nutrients in the soil, the rise of processed and calorie-dense foods, and the potential impacts of synthetic chemicals in the food supply. Together, these environmental and dietary factors offer important insight into how the modern food environment may be influencing the broader health challenges of our time.

Soil Depletion and Nutrient Deficiency

The nutritional quality of the food we eat begins long before it reaches our plate. It starts in the soil.

Healthy soil is more than just dirt, it is a living, dynamic system rich in organic matter, minerals, and microorganisms that make nutrients available to plants. For most of human history, crops were grown in soils that were naturally replenished through composting, seasonal rotation, and biodiversity. These traditional practices allowed fruits, vegetables, and grains to absorb a wide range of minerals and trace elements, which were then passed along the food chain to animals and humans.

But over the past several decades, industrial agriculture has significantly changed the way soil is managed. Intensive farming techniques, such as monoculture cropping, synthetic fertilizers, and chemical pesticides, have increased yields in the short term, but often at the cost of long-term soil health. Continuous planting without allowing the land to rest, combined with the loss of organic inputs, has led to a widespread decline in soil mineral content and microbial diversity.

This loss has measurable effects. According to a widely cited study published in the *Journal of the American College of Nutrition*, researchers found that between 1950 and 1999, the nutrient content of 43 garden crops in the U.S. had significantly declined. On average, vegetables showed reductions of up to 38% in key nutrients such as calcium, magnesium, potassium, and iron. Similar findings have been reported in the United Kingdom and Canada, where soil mineral depletion is also impacting food quality.

This means that even when individuals consume what appear to be healthy, plant-rich diets, they may not be receiving the same concentration of nutrients that earlier generations once did. The apple or spinach on today's table may look similar to what was served 70 years ago, but its micronutrient profile can be noticeably diminished.

Beyond mineral loss, modern farming practices also disrupt the balance of life within the soil itself. The overuse of herbicides and synthetic nitrogen fertilizers can reduce populations of beneficial microorganisms, tiny bacteria and fungi that help plants break down organic material and absorb minerals more efficiently. Without this microbial support system, crops may grow in appearance but remain nutritionally shallow beneath the surface.

While the implications of nutrient decline are still being studied, public health experts and agricultural scientists are increasingly voicing concern. Food is not just about calories, it is about the invisible compounds that help the body function smoothly: enzymes, cofactors, antioxidants, and trace minerals. When these are missing or diminished, the body may struggle to maintain its balance and perform at its best, even in the absence of hunger or illness.

In short, the health of the soil is inseparable from the quality of the food it produces. And as the soil becomes depleted, so too does the nutritional foundation of our meals. Recognizing this connection is an important first step in understanding how large-scale environmental changes can influence our most personal measure of health—what we put in our bodies every day.

Modern Food: High in Calories, Low in Nutrients

In today's food landscape, convenience often comes at a cost. As the pace of daily life accelerates, so too does the demand for fast, affordable, and long-lasting food. In response, the global food industry has turned increasingly to industrial processing techniques, producing items that are calorie-dense, shelf-stable, and engineered for taste. While these foods are widely available and easy to prepare, concerns continue to rise over what they offer nutritionally, and, just as importantly, what they may lack.

Many of these foods rely heavily on refined carbohydrates, added sugars, industrial seed oils, and synthetic additives. Though they can satisfy cravings and offer a familiar sensory experience, they often contain limited amounts of essential nutrients such as vitamins, minerals, and fiber. This class of foods, frequently referred to as "ultra-processed", now accounts for over half of total caloric intake in many industrialized countries, including the United States.

The issue is not just one of excessive calories; it's about nutritional dilution. When diets consist mostly of nutrient-poor foods, a paradox can emerge: people may consume more than enough food to meet energy needs while still falling short in the micronutrients necessary to support their body's daily functions. This phenomenon, often described by public health researchers as being "overfed but undernourished," has become increasingly common in high-income countries.

Data from the U.S. Department of Agriculture (USDA) and the National Health and Nutrition Examination Survey (NHANES) consistently show that large portions of the population fall short of the recommended intake for key nutrients. For example, more than 90% of Americans consume less fiber than recommended. Other commonly under-consumed nutrients include magnesium, vitamin

E, potassium, and choline, each important for normal physiological function.

Part of the problem lies in the engineered nature of many processed foods. Designed to optimize taste and texture, they often contain combinations of sugar, salt, and fat that encourage habitual consumption. Over time, this can lead to a gradual shift away from more nutrient-dense whole foods. While any single food product may be harmless in moderation, long-term reliance on these options can reduce overall dietary quality, leaving individuals with fewer protective nutrients than intended.

In addition to nutrient gaps, there is growing public attention on the widespread use of synthetic compounds in processed food manufacturing. Additives such as preservatives, sweeteners, colorants, emulsifiers, and stabilizers are commonly used to enhance shelf life, flavor, and appearance. While these substances are approved for use by regulatory agencies and are generally recognized as safe within set limits, questions remain about the potential long-term impact of frequent, cumulative exposure, especially when consumed daily over many years.

Artificial sweeteners, for example, are commonly found in diet beverages and low-sugar products. While they serve as a sugar substitute, some researchers continue to explore how they may interact with metabolism or digestive balance. Preservatives like

BHA and BHT are added to cereals and snacks to prevent spoilage but have been the subject of scientific review and consumer debate. Artificial food dyes such as Red 40 and Yellow 5, used in many candies, drinks, and children's snacks, have been banned or restricted in some countries based on public pressure and precautionary standards, despite remaining approved in the U.S.

Emulsifiers like polysorbate 80 and carboxymethylcellulose, used in ice creams, sauces, and dressings, are also undergoing continued research to better understand their effects on digestion and gut ecology. Though current regulations support their safety at defined levels, the broader nutritional conversation now extends beyond individual ingredients, toward the overall dietary pattern and its long-term implications.

In many households, ultra-processed foods are not occasional indulgences but form the bulk of daily meals. This has created a nutritional environment in which many people are consuming more calories and more additives than any previous generation, often without realizing how much their food has changed in composition and origin.

This shift raises an important question for the modern era: in a world of technological advancement and food abundance, are we truly nourishing our bodies? Or simply fueling them?

The Role of Pesticides and Chemical Exposure

Modern agriculture has become increasingly dependent on synthetic chemicals to meet the demands of large-scale food production. Pesticides, herbicides, antibiotics, and growth hormones are widely used to increase yield, prevent crop damage, and optimize livestock growth. While these chemicals have contributed to higher efficiency and food availability, growing public concern now centers on how continued exposure to these substances may affect long-term health and food quality.

Pesticides, including insecticides, herbicides, and fungicides, are applied to billions of acres of crops each year. According to data from the U.S. Environmental Protection Agency (EPA), over 1 billion pounds of pesticides are used annually in the United States alone. Globally, that figure exceeds 5 billion pounds per year. These chemicals are designed to disrupt biological processes in pests, but some may remain on food crops and enter the human food supply. The U.S. Department of Agriculture (USDA) regularly tests for pesticide residues on foods and reports that a majority of conventionally grown produce contains detectable levels of at least one residue, even after washing and peeling.

The herbicide glyphosate, for example, is among the most widely used agricultural chemicals in the world. It is commonly sprayed on genetically modified crops like corn and soy, as well as non-GMO crops such as oats and wheat shortly before harvest. While glyphosate has been reviewed and approved for use by agencies such as the EPA and the European Food Safety Authority (EFSA), some international organizations, including the International Agency for Research on Cancer (IARC), have classified it as a "probable human carcinogen" based on limited human evidence and sufficient evidence from animal studies. This divergence in regulatory classification has fueled public debate and prompted further investigation into its long-term effects, especially in relation to cumulative exposure through food and water.

In addition to crop-related chemicals, antibiotics and growth hormones are commonly used in industrial livestock operations. In the United States, data from the Food and Drug Administration (FDA) shows that approximately 65–70% of medically important antibiotics sold each year are used in animal agriculture, primarily to promote growth and prevent disease in crowded feedlot conditions. Public health organizations, including the Centers for Disease Control and Prevention (CDC), have warned that this widespread use may contribute to the development of antibiotic-resistant bacteria, a growing threat to global health systems. While regulatory limits are in place for antibiotic residues in meat and dairy, the broader concern is how frequent low-level exposure may affect microbial balance over time.

Hormones such as recombinant bovine growth hormone (rBGH) are still used in some dairy production systems to increase milk output. Although the U.S. FDA considers rBGH safe for use, the

European Union and Canada have banned it due to animal welfare concerns and ongoing debates over potential health implications. These differing regulatory stances reflect both scientific uncertainty and varying national approaches to risk management.

Beyond individual substances, researchers are increasingly examining the cumulative effect of chemical exposures over a lifetime. Many people consume trace amounts of multiple substances daily, pesticide residues from produce, preservatives from packaged foods, and hormones or antibiotics from animal products. While each chemical may fall within approved limits, questions remain about how these exposures interact in the body over time, especially in sensitive populations such as children, pregnant women, or those with underlying health conditions.

This growing body of research has led to increasing consumer demand for transparency in food production. Surveys conducted by the Pew Research Center and other institutions show that a majority of consumers express concern over pesticide use in farming and prefer to have more information about how their food is produced. In response, organic and chemical-free farming methods are gaining traction, not only as environmental practices but also as consumer choices driven by the desire to minimize unnecessary exposure to synthetic compounds.

In short, the role of agricultural chemicals in the modern food system is complex. While these tools serve essential functions in protecting crops and livestock, the public health conversation is shifting. It now includes not only the safety of individual substances at regulated doses, but the long-term effects of combined, low-level exposure across many years. As scientific inquiry continues, awareness of chemical inputs, both visible and invisible, remains an important part of understanding how food choices intersect with broader wellness concerns.

Mental and Emotional Well-Being: A Global Challenge

Health is more than the absence of physical symptoms; it includes the emotional and psychological resilience that allows individuals to cope with life's challenges. Yet around the world, mental health concerns are rising at an alarming pace, affecting people of all ages, backgrounds, and communities.

According to the World Health Organization (WHO), more than 264 million people worldwide experience depression, and this number has been steadily increasing in recent years. Alongside depression, anxiety disorders and chronic stress-related conditions are now recognized as major contributors to the global burden of disease. While many factors influence mental health, including genetics, environment, trauma, and socioeconomic circumstances, modern life presents unique pressures that appear to be contributing to growing psychological strain.

In particular, urban environments have been associated with increased levels of stress and emotional exhaustion. Fast-paced living, digital overstimulation, financial instability, and social disconnection can combine to erode mental well-being over time. The COVID-19 pandemic further intensified these challenges, placing millions under prolonged isolation, uncertainty, and disruption, all of which can contribute to feelings of anxiety, hopelessness, or burnout.

The mental health crisis is not limited to adults. Adolescents and young adults are now facing unprecedented emotional demands. The Centers for Disease Control and Prevention (CDC) reports that 44% of high school students experienced persistent feelings of sadness or hopelessness in 2021, up from 26% in 2009. The same report found that 22% of students had seriously considered suicide within the past year, and 10% had made an attempt, with particularly high rates among females and LGBTQ+ youth. These numbers are deeply concerning and reflect the growing vulnerability of younger generations as they navigate academic pressures, social media, identity formation, and often a lack of stable support systems.

Even among adults, data shows that millions live with undiagnosed or untreated mental health challenges. According to the National

Institute of Mental Health (NIMH), more than 1 in 5 U.S. adults, roughly 58 million people, experience mental illness each year. These numbers do not include those who may struggle silently, without formal diagnosis or access to care.

The mind-body connection is a vital but often overlooked aspect of health. While mental health is complex and influenced by many factors, researchers have increasingly explored how lifestyle patterns, such as sleep quality, physical activity, nutrition, and chronic stress levels, can affect emotional resilience and cognitive function. Poor sleep, for instance, has been associated with changes in mood regulation, energy levels, and focus. Sedentary behavior and nutrient-poor diets are also being studied for their role in supporting or undermining overall mental well-being.

Chronic stress, in particular, plays a unique role. When the body's stress response is activated frequently, without sufficient time to recover, it may impact systems involved in energy metabolism, focus, and even immune regulation. While scientific understanding is still evolving, a growing number of studies suggest that supporting mental health requires a holistic view of overall wellness, rather than compartmentalizing physical and psychological care.

Despite the growing recognition of mental health as a global priority, access to care remains limited in many regions. Stigma, lack of resources, and insufficient support systems continue to prevent many individuals from seeking help. At the same time, increasing public awareness is shifting the narrative, making it more acceptable to talk about mental health, to share challenges, and to seek out strategies that promote emotional well-being.

Mental health is not just a medical issue; it's a human one. And in a world that often demands constant performance, productivity, and perfection, it's more important than ever to create space for rest, reflection, and connection. Recognizing the scope of the mental health crisis is not a sign of despair, it is the first step toward rebuilding the foundations of psychological wellness in modern life.

When Conventional Care Feels Incomplete

Conventional medicine has made extraordinary advancements in treating infections, managing trauma, and extending life expectancy through emergency care and surgical interventions. In acute care situations, such as heart attacks, injuries, or infectious disease outbreaks, conventional approaches remain irreplaceable and often lifesaving.

However, when it comes to the long-term management of chronic health conditions, such as hypertension, type 2 diabetes, and autoimmune disorders, the strengths of conventional medicine may not always align with the needs of patients seeking sustainable well-being. Many chronic illnesses unfold gradually, with roots in daily lifestyle patterns, environmental exposures, and systemic imbalances. In such cases, an approach focused primarily on symptom management, often through lifelong medication, may not address the broader context in which the illness developed.

In the United States, 6 in 10 adults live with at least one chronic disease, and 4 in 10 have two or more, according to the Centers for Disease Control and Prevention (CDC). These conditions, ranging from cardiovascular issues to metabolic dysfunction, are now the leading drivers of healthcare costs, accounting for over 90% of the nation's $4.5 trillion in annual health expenditures. Much of this spending is directed toward pharmaceuticals and procedures aimed at managing symptoms rather than restoring underlying balance.

Medications play a vital role in helping patients stabilize their conditions, and for many, they are essential. However, there is growing awareness that pharmaceuticals, while effective in controlling indicators like blood pressure, glucose levels, or cholesterol, may not always reverse the broader physiological changes contributing to illness. This creates a model of care that is highly reactive, focused on managing flare-ups and lab values, rather than preventive or restorative.

For instance, a person diagnosed with high blood pressure may be prescribed antihypertensive medication, yet may not receive in-depth support for dietary changes, stress reduction, or physical activity, factors that public health research has shown to be significant contributors to cardiovascular health. Similarly, individuals with insulin resistance may receive glucose-lowering drugs, but less personalized guidance on sleep, movement, and nutrition, which could play a role in improving metabolic resilience.

Pharmaceuticals also come with potential side effects. While all medications approved by regulatory bodies undergo safety evaluations, real-world use often reveals additional risks, especially when prescriptions are used over long periods or in combination. For example, long-term use of non-steroidal anti-inflammatory drugs (NSAIDs) has been associated in some studies with increased risk of gastrointestinal bleeding and kidney strain. Mental health medications, such as antidepressants or anti-anxiety drugs, have helped many individuals, but can also bring challenges related to dosage changes, withdrawal, and side effects such as fatigue or emotional blunting.

Another example that has drawn public interest is the use of statin drugs to lower cholesterol. Statins are among the most commonly prescribed medications in the world and are considered a cornerstone of cardiovascular risk management. However, some studies have raised questions about whether statins may reduce levels of coenzyme Q10 (CoQ10), a naturally occurring compound involved in cellular energy production. While the clinical significance of this effect is still under debate, it highlights the complexity of modifying one biomarker without considering the broader metabolic network it influences.

It's important to note that healthcare providers are increasingly aware of these dynamics. Many doctors now integrate lifestyle recommendations into care plans, and interest in integrative and functional medicine is growing across mainstream institutions. Nonetheless, systemic constraints, such as time-limited appointments, insurance coding models, and limited access to nutrition and wellness specialists, can make it difficult for patients to receive truly comprehensive care within conventional frameworks.

The result is that many individuals find themselves on multiple medications, managing their symptoms but not necessarily improving their long-term vitality. This has sparked a wider conversation: what does it mean to truly support health?

Rather than positioning pharmaceuticals and holistic approaches in opposition, a growing movement is calling for collaboration, a model in which symptom management is paired with root-cause exploration, and where the body's natural capacity for resilience is supported alongside medical treatment. By shifting the focus from short-term control to long-term optimization, the future of medicine may become not only more effective, but more empowering.

Limitations of Synthetic Supplements

For decades, multivitamins have been marketed as a simple, convenient solution to fill dietary gaps and maintain overall health. In fact, multivitamin use is so common that more than one-third of all U.S. adults report taking one regularly, according to data from the National Institutes of Health (NIH). Yet despite their popularity, recent research has raised important questions about the long-term effectiveness and safety of synthetic multivitamin formulations.

Large-scale studies have not consistently shown benefits from multivitamin use in the prevention of chronic diseases. For example, the Physicians' Health Study II, one of the largest randomized trials involving over 14,000 male physicians, found no significant reduction in major cardiovascular events or overall mortality from multivitamin use over more than a decade of follow-up. Similarly, a meta-analysis published in the journal *Annals of Internal Medicine* in 2013 concluded that most multivitamins do not reduce the risk of heart disease, cancer, or cognitive decline and may not offer meaningful benefit for the general population.

In some cases, concerns have been raised about potential downsides. A study published in the *Archives of Internal Medicine* in 2011 tracked over 38,000 older women and found an association, not causation, between certain supplement combinations, including multivitamins, and a slightly increased risk of mortality. While further studies are needed to understand these findings in context, they challenge the assumption that more supplementation automatically leads to better health.

Beyond the lack of clear preventive benefit, some healthcare professionals and researchers are beginning to explore the impact of long-term use of isolated synthetic vitamins, especially at high doses. Excessive intake of fat-soluble vitamins such as A, D, and E, especially in their synthetic forms, can accumulate in body tissues and may lead to adverse effects if not properly metabolized. Though rare, cases of vitamin toxicity have been documented, including hypervitaminosis A, which can impact liver function, and vitamin D toxicity, which can alter calcium balance in the body.

Another point of concern involves the formulation and origin of many synthetic vitamins. While legally safe for consumption in approved doses, most synthetic vitamins are produced in laboratories using chemical processes that replicate the structure of natural nutrients, but often exclude the complex network of enzymes, coenzymes, and phytochemicals that accompany vitamins in whole foods. For example, synthetic vitamin E (dl-alpha-tocopherol) differs structurally from the natural form and may not be as efficiently utilized by the body. Similarly, some forms of synthetic folic acid require multiple metabolic steps to become bioactive, which can be less efficient in certain individuals with genetic variations (such as MTHFR mutations).

The bioavailability of synthetic nutrients, how easily they are absorbed and used by the body, can vary widely based on both the form of the vitamin and the individual's digestive and metabolic function. Some studies suggest that nutrients derived from whole-food sources, which contain the full spectrum of naturally occurring cofactors and enzymes, may be more easily recognized and utilized by the body, especially in those with compromised digestion or chronic inflammation.

That's why in *The Medicine-Free, Illness-Free Series*, we emphasize food-first and food-based supplementation where possible. While synthetic multivitamins may serve a purpose in certain medical contexts or for individuals with specific deficiencies, many people may benefit more from nutrient-dense diets supported by whole-food-based formulas that provide vitamins and minerals in their natural matrix.

This is not about creating fear around synthetic supplements. Rather, it's about encouraging a shift in how we view nutrition, from "pill for every gap" convenience toward nutritional integrity, where the body receives its nourishment in forms it has evolved to digest and utilize over thousands of years.

As always, supplement decisions should be made in consultation with qualified health professionals who can evaluate your unique nutritional needs. And while no supplement replaces a healthy lifestyle, the form and quality of your nutrients do matter and they can play a powerful role in how effectively your body functions and feels every day.

Why Natural Health is the Future

The world is facing a turning point in health. Chronic illnesses have become more widespread than ever, shaped by modern lifestyles, processed diets, environmental exposures, and stress-heavy routines. At the same time, many people are discovering that conventional medicine, while extraordinarily effective for trauma, emergencies, and acute care, often lacks a sustainable approach to long-term wellness and resilience.

According to the Centers for Disease Control and Prevention (CDC), 6 in 10 U.S. adults live with a chronic disease, and 4 in 10 live with two or more. These numbers continue to rise despite record-breaking healthcare spending, which topped $4.5 trillion in the U.S. in 2022 alone. Globally, chronic conditions are now the leading cause of death and disability, prompting individuals, practitioners, and policymakers to look beyond short-term symptom relief toward more comprehensive, root-level care.

This growing awareness has fueled interest in natural health, a diverse and evidence-informed field that emphasizes balance, prevention, and the body's innate capacity for self-regulation. Rooted in centuries of traditional wisdom and increasingly supported by modern science, natural therapies such as herbal medicine, nutritional therapy, acupuncture, grounding, breathwork, and mind-body practices are gaining renewed attention for their ability to support whole-person wellness.

Unlike conventional approaches that often center on managing specific symptoms or lab values, natural health looks at the broader picture: how nutrition, lifestyle, emotions, sleep, environment, and energy patterns interact to shape long-term vitality. While natural therapies do not replace emergency care or necessary prescriptions, they offer a complementary path, one that empowers individuals to take a more active role in their daily health.

The shift toward natural health is not just a personal preference; it is becoming a global movement. The World Health Organization (WHO) recognizes the value of traditional and complementary medicine and has called for its integration into national health systems. In the United States, surveys from the National Center for Complementary and Integrative Health (NCCIH) show that nearly 1 in 3 adults now uses some form of complementary or alternative therapy, ranging from herbal supplements and meditation to acupuncture and yoga.

This rise reflects more than a search for alternatives, it reflects a desire for personalized, patient-centered care that acknowledges the connection between body, mind, and environment. As people become increasingly aware of how stress, toxins, inactivity, and poor nutrition affect their well-being, they are turning toward approaches that feel aligned with their values, their rhythms, and their goals.

This chapter explores why natural therapies are gaining momentum in today's healthcare landscape. It will highlight their role in addressing underlying contributors to illness, supporting prevention, reducing side effect burden, and promoting long-term vitality. As the world becomes more complex, and the limits of symptom-centered care become more visible, natural health offers a timely invitation: to think differently, live more consciously, and engage in proactive, integrated care that honors the whole person.

The Rise of Natural Health: Global and US Trends

Over the past decade, natural health has shifted from a niche interest to a global movement. Driven by increased access to information, evolving values, and a growing desire for preventive, whole-person care, millions of people are turning to holistic solutions as part of their daily health routine. What was once viewed as complementary is now becoming central to how individuals define and pursue wellness.

Market Expansion: A Shift from Steady Growth to Rapid Acceleration

In both the United States and globally, the complementary and alternative medicine (CAM) sector is experiencing rapid growth, far outpacing past projections and signaling a shift in healthcare priorities.

United States Market Trends

2018 to 2023: The U.S. Complementary and Alternative Medicine (CAM) market expanded from $14.8 billion in 2018 to $28.1 billion in 2023, reflecting a Compound Annual Growth Rate (CAGR) of approximately 13.9% during this period (Grand View Research, 2024).

2024 to 2030: Forecasts predict that the U.S. CAM market will grow from $28.1 billion in 2023 to $124.2 billion by 2030, with an anticipated CAGR of 23.9% (Grand View Research, 2024).

Global Market Trends

2018 to 2023: The global CAM market grew from $82.27 billion in 2018 to $144.68 billion in 2023, representing a CAGR of approximately 11.9% (Grand View Research, 2024).

2024 to 2030: Analysts project that the market will accelerate dramatically, expanding from $144.68 billion in 2023 to $694.22 billion by 2030, with a projected CAGR of 25.1% (Grand View Research, 2024; Research and Markets, 2024).

This growth reflects a broader rethinking of what health support should look like, moving beyond pharmaceutical-only models to include sustainable, individualized, and minimally invasive therapies.

Consumer Adoption Rates: A Growing Movement Toward Holistic Health

Consumer behavior is evolving alongside these market trends. In 2021, approximately 24% of U.S. adults reported using herbal medicines, supplements, or teas to support their health (*Statista, 2021*). Just a year later, that number jumped to 36.7%, with individuals engaging in practices such as acupuncture, meditation, yoga, and nutritional supplementation (*National Center for Complementary and Integrative Health, 2022*).

This growing interest is not simply about trying something new, it represents a shift in how people engage with their well-being. Rather than waiting for illness to develop, many are choosing a proactive, wellness-oriented lifestyle that incorporates natural therapies into daily habits.

What's Driving the Rise of Natural Health?

Several converging forces are fueling this shift.

Access to Information: The digital age has empowered individuals to research therapies, understand their options, and make more informed decisions about their health. As consumers become more health-literate, they increasingly explore natural methods of support alongside or in place of conventional approaches.

Awareness of Side Effects: While conventional medicine plays a vital role in many health scenarios, growing awareness of potential long-term medication side effects has led many to seek gentler strategies, especially for chronic conditions. Individuals are exploring alternatives that align with their desire for fewer adverse reactions and more holistic care.

The Rise of Preventive Wellness: People are redefining health as something to be actively cultivated, not just repaired when lost. This shift is leading to increased adoption of nutrition, herbal support, acupuncture, mind-body techniques, and other practices that focus on system-wide balance and resilience.

Environmental and Ethical Values: Modern consumers increasingly care about how their health choices affect the planet. Clean ingredients, sustainable farming, and transparent sourcing matter, leading more people to choose organic supplements, plant-based remedies, and whole-food products that reflect their ethical standards.

A Paradigm Shift in Healthcare Priorities

The rise of natural health is more than a trend; it marks a deeper cultural movement. Patients are no longer satisfied with symptom-focused care alone. Instead, they seek personalized, integrative strategies that consider the full picture of health: physical, mental, emotional, environmental, and even spiritual.

Healthcare professionals are taking notice. Medical schools are beginning to offer courses in integrative medicine, and hospital systems across the U.S. are incorporating complementary therapies like nutrition counseling, acupuncture, and mindfulness into their treatment offerings.

As this momentum continues, natural health is poised to play an increasingly central role in the future of healthcare, offering not a replacement, but a partner in the broader effort to support lifelong well-being.

Root-Cause Care: A Smarter Approach to Long-Term Wellness

One of the most meaningful differences between conventional and natural approaches to health lies in the focus on root causes. Rather than concentrating solely on immediate symptom relief, many natural health practices aim to explore and support the deeper factors that may be contributing to imbalance in the body. This shift in perspective is especially relevant today, as more individuals face ongoing health challenges that are influenced by lifestyle, environment, and daily habits.

Conventional medicine has proven extraordinarily effective in managing acute conditions, such as infections, injuries, and emergencies. However, for long-term conditions, like persistent fatigue, digestive discomfort, or metabolic imbalances, patients often find themselves in a cycle of symptom management, returning frequently for new prescriptions or dose adjustments. These strategies may stabilize symptoms, but they may not fully address the systemic patterns that led to the condition in the first place.

In contrast, many natural health systems take a broader view. They look beyond the presenting symptoms to examine how nutrition, stress, sleep, movement, toxin exposure, and emotional health might be interacting to influence well-being. This functional or systems-based lens does not oppose conventional treatment but complements it by helping patients explore the context of their symptoms and make informed, personalized adjustments.

Take, for example, an individual dealing with elevated blood pressure. In a conventional setting, medication may be prescribed to control the numbers, which can be essential in high-risk cases. In a natural health setting, however, a practitioner may also explore dietary sodium intake, mineral status (such as potassium or magnesium), stress resilience, hydration, and sleep quality, all of which can influence cardiovascular function. The goal is not to replace medication, but to offer a more comprehensive understanding of how daily choices shape long-term outcomes.

Similarly, for those experiencing recurring joint discomfort or muscle tension, over-the-counter pain relievers like NSAIDs can provide short-term relief. Yet frequent reliance on these solutions may mask deeper patterns, such as inflammatory dietary triggers, postural strain, or micronutrient deficiencies. Natural approaches may include gentle movement, anti-inflammatory herbs, nutritional support, or stress-reduction techniques to reduce the frequency and intensity of discomfort over time.

This focus on root-cause support is especially valuable in addressing chronic lifestyle-related issues. According to the CDC, many of the most common chronic conditions, including heart concerns, metabolic disorders, and mood imbalances, are influenced by modifiable factors like diet, exercise, and stress management. Natural health practitioners often begin here, guiding individuals to make sustainable, empowering changes that support the body's normal regulatory functions.

While natural therapies do not promise instant results, they often foster a collaborative approach to health, inviting individuals to explore the "why" behind recurring patterns and participate actively in their wellness journey. This can lead not only to better symptom management but also to a renewed sense of connection with one's body, energy, and life goals.

Whole-Food and Nature Solutions: A Fundamental Shift

For decades, synthetic multivitamins and isolated nutrients have been promoted as a convenient way to "fill nutritional gaps" and support overall wellness. However, large-scale studies have questioned the long-term effectiveness of synthetic supplementation, and in some cases, raised concerns about potential downsides, especially when used in high doses or without medical oversight.

Whole-food-based solutions offer a different approach. Instead of isolated, lab-created compounds, they deliver nutrients in their natural form, alongside essential cofactors, enzymes, and plant compounds that help optimize absorption and function. These nutrient-rich sources are more easily recognized and utilized by the body, offering a way to support wellness and long-term nutritional balance in alignment with how the body has evolved to process food.

Whole-Food Nutrition: How Nature Delivers What the Body Truly Needs

At the heart of many natural healing systems is a deceptively simple principle: the body recognizes and responds best to nutrients in their natural, whole-food form. Rather than relying on synthetic vitamins or heavily fortified processed products, whole-food-based nutrition provides what the body has evolved to use—real nutrients, embedded in their natural matrix of enzymes, cofactors, and phytochemicals.

Research supports this idea. For example:

A 2012 meta-analysis published in *Advances in Nutrition* found that nutrients consumed from whole foods often have higher bioavailability and greater synergistic effects than isolated synthetic forms. In whole foods, vitamins are accompanied by fiber, antioxidants, trace minerals, and other naturally occurring compounds that enhance absorption and modulate how the nutrients function in the body.

Studies comparing synthetic vs. natural Vitamin E (dl-alpha-tocopherol vs. d-alpha-tocopherol) consistently show that the natural form is up to two times more bioavailable, meaning it remains longer in circulation and is more efficiently retained by tissues (NIH Office of Dietary Supplements, 2021).

Natural folate from leafy greens and legumes is absorbed and utilized differently than synthetic folic acid, which must undergo enzymatic conversion in the liver. Individuals with MTHFR gene variants (estimated to affect up to 40% of the population) may have reduced ability to process synthetic folic acid effectively, making whole-food folate sources a more biologically compatible option.

Why Isolated Nutrients Fall Short

Synthetic vitamins are typically created in labs from petrochemical or industrial fermentation processes. While they may match the molecular structure of naturally occurring vitamins, they lack the supportive compounds, like polyphenols, enzymes, or mineral co-factors, that exist in real food. Without these, absorption and activation in the body can be limited or uneven.

Furthermore, many synthetic multivitamins deliver unnaturally high doses of nutrients in isolated form. When consumed in excess or without proper balance, these can act more like drugs than food, potentially creating imbalances rather than restoring them. For example:

Excess synthetic Vitamin A (retinyl palmitate) has been associated with liver stress and bone density issues in long-term supplementation studies.

Synthetic beta-carotene supplements, when given to smokers in high doses, were shown in a 1996 study (*NEJM*) to actually increase lung cancer risk, a result not seen when beta-carotene is consumed from fruits and vegetables.

Whole-food-based supplements avoid this issue by delivering nutrients in physiological, not pharmacological, doses, and always in the presence of their natural cofactors.

Examples of Powerful Whole-Food-Based Solutions

Natural health practices often center around whole-food sources that provide therapeutic benefits without the need for synthetic additives or mega-doses. Here are a few examples integrated across *The Medicine-Free, Illness-Free Series*:

Organ Meats (Animal Organ Therapy): Rich in naturally occurring fat-soluble vitamins (A, D, E, K), B-complex vitamins, iron, zinc, and bioactive peptides that support cellular and hormonal function. Research shows that organ meats are among the most nutrient-dense foods available per calorie, yet are almost absent from modern diets.

Medicinal Mushrooms (Mushroom Therapy): Contain beta-glucans, ergothioneine, and triterpenoids, compounds shown in animal and in-vitro studies to support immune modulation, antioxidant defense, and stress resilience. Shiitake, Reishi, Lion's Mane, and Cordyceps are among the most researched.

Amino Acid-Rich Foods (Amino Acid Therapy): Bone broth, collagen, and fermented protein sources deliver glycine, glutamine, and proline, essential for gut integrity, neurotransmitter balance, and tissue repair. These amino acids are difficult to obtain in meaningful amounts from processed diets.

Herbal Preparations (Herbal Therapy): Many herbs contain unique phytochemicals that interact with human enzymes and receptors in subtle, adaptive ways. For example, turmeric curcumin, astragalus polysaccharides, and licorice flavonoids have each been studied for their effects on inflammatory markers and cellular stress responses in both preclinical and clinical settings.

Whole Foods (HOPED Protocol): These support the gut microbiome and deliver prebiotics, short-chain fatty acids, and naturally occurring probiotics. Research shows that microbiome diversity is closely associated with immune, metabolic, and even emotional resilience.

Why This Matters in Today's World

Modern diets, despite being calorie-rich, are often nutrient-poor, filled with ultra-processed foods that lack fiber, antioxidants, and trace minerals. The CDC reports that over 90% of U.S. adults fall short on key nutrients such as fiber, potassium, magnesium, and vitamins A, C, D, and E. Meanwhile, the rise in chronic conditions, from metabolic stress to low immunity, points to a system in need of deeper nourishment, not just short-term fixes.

Whole-food-based natural solutions don't just fill a gap; they rebuild a foundation. By supplying nutrients in their full-spectrum form and supporting systems like detoxification, immunity, and digestion, they help create the conditions in which the body can self-regulate and maintain balance.

Gentle on Your Body

One of the reasons many people are turning to natural therapies is their reputation for being gentler on the body. While conventional medicine plays a vital role in managing serious and acute conditions, it often involves pharmaceutical interventions that, by design, strongly influence biochemical pathways. These medications can be life-saving, but they also frequently come with a long list of potential side effects, ranging from mild digestive discomfort to more serious complications, especially when used long term or in combination with other drugs.

According to the U.S. Department of Health and Human Services, adverse drug reactions account for more than 1.3 million emergency room visits and approximately 350,000 hospitalizations in the United States each year. The FDA's Adverse Event Reporting System (FAERS) continues to document side effects linked to commonly used medications, including everything from blood pressure drugs and antidepressants to cholesterol-lowering statins. As medical care becomes increasingly complex, especially in older populations or those with multiple chronic conditions, these risks become harder to ignore.

In contrast, natural therapies are often chosen for their low side-effect profile and long history of traditional use. Rather than overwhelming the body with high-potency compounds, these therapies aim to work in cooperation with the body's normal rhythms and regulatory systems. Many people report feeling supported, rather than suppressed, when using natural solutions such as herbal infusions, whole-food-based supplements, or lifestyle-based practices like breathwork and grounding. These approaches are not only non-invasive but are often seen as sustainable because they can be used consistently without producing the cumulative side effects often seen with pharmaceuticals.

Consider turmeric, a spice long used in traditional medicine and now studied for its active compound curcumin. Research suggests that curcumin may help maintain inflammatory balance in the body. While it is not a replacement for anti-inflammatory drugs in serious medical conditions, it has shown promise in supporting joint comfort and immune health without the same digestive risks commonly associated with non-steroidal anti-inflammatory drugs (NSAIDs). Similarly, magnesium supplementation, when used appropriately, has been shown to support sleep quality, muscle relaxation, and stress recovery with minimal side effects, most commonly mild digestive upset when taken in high doses.

This gentle approach makes natural therapies especially appealing for individuals who are sensitive to medications, have multiple health concerns, or are simply seeking long-term wellness strategies that align with a lifestyle of prevention and balance. Because many natural therapies do not rely on synthetic compounds or pharmaceutical mechanisms, they often carry a lower risk of interactions, making them an option that can be tailored over time as a person's health evolves.

That said, natural does not always mean risk-free. Herbs, supplements, and even food-based remedies may interact with medications or affect people differently depending on their unique physiology. Responsible use, including guidance from trained health professionals, ensures that natural therapies are used appropriately and safely, particularly when integrated into an existing treatment plan.

When thoughtfully applied, natural health strategies offer something increasingly valuable in today's complex medical environment: the opportunity to support health with fewer unwanted effects. Rather than forcing a single mechanism of change, these approaches help create the conditions for the body to balance, adapt, and thrive, gently and sustainably.

Personalized and Patient-Centered Care

One of the most powerful reasons people are turning to natural health is the deeply personalized approach it offers. Rather than applying a one-size-fits-all model, many natural therapies emphasize care that is tailored to the individual, considering their unique biology, lifestyle, emotional health, and environmental exposures. This philosophy aligns with a growing realization across the healthcare industry: personalization is no longer a luxury but a necessity.

While conventional medicine excels in acute care, it often operates within time-limited appointments and standardized treatment protocols designed for population-level efficiency. These approaches are critical for public health and emergency medicine, but they may not always meet the needs of individuals navigating complex, chronic, or lifestyle-related concerns. Natural therapies, by contrast, begin by asking: what makes this person unique, and what support do they truly need?

This desire for individualized care is not just a theory. According to a 2022 survey by the National Institutes of Health and Health Affairs, 85% of patients say they want their care to reflect their personal circumstances, values, and preferences, not just a diagnosis. Many people are looking for care that considers their story, not just their symptoms.

Traditional Chinese Medicine (TCM) offers a clear example of what this looks like in practice. In TCM, treatment is never based solely on a disease name. Practitioners consider the person as a whole, evaluating signs like digestion, energy flow, sleep, emotions, tongue characteristics, and even sensitivity to climate. Two patients with the same diagnosis might receive completely different herbal formulas or acupuncture protocols, depending on their unique constitution.

This patient-centered focus is what makes TCM both highly adaptive and deeply rooted in real-world human diversity.

This principle extends into modern integrative and functional medicine as well. Today, practitioners increasingly use advanced tools such as genetic testing, hormone panels, and microbiome analysis to help guide lifestyle and nutrition strategies. This mirrors trends in the broader medical field, particularly the U.S. Precision Medicine Initiative, which emphasizes the use of genetic, lifestyle, and environmental data to make care more individualized and effective.

Nutrition science has also embraced this shift. The global personalized nutrition market, which includes microbiome-driven diet plans and supplement protocols based on DNA or blood biomarkers, was valued at over $8 billion in 2020 and is projected to exceed $16 billion by 2027. Consumers are no longer satisfied with generic diet plans, they want recommendations that match their body, their metabolism, and their goals.

This personalized model of care also fosters deeper engagement between practitioner and patient. Studies published in *BMJ* and the *Journal of General Internal Medicine* report that the average primary care visit in the U.S. lasts just 15 to 18 minutes. In contrast, natural health consultations, whether in TCM, integrative nutrition, or functional medicine, often last 45 minutes to an hour or more. This extended time allows for meaningful listening, thoughtful assessment, and collaborative planning, which many patients find empowering and reassuring.

Personalized care also means recognizing the role of emotional well-being in physical health. Natural health systems often explore how stress, trauma, and belief patterns may influence healing. This level of inquiry is not always addressed in fast-paced clinical settings but is fundamental to many holistic frameworks. When people feel seen, heard, and understood, and not just treated, they are more likely to engage fully in their wellness journey.

As the world moves toward more individualized, whole-person care models, natural therapies offer a long-standing example of how this can work. They don't just customize based on symptoms; they customize based on the full complexity of human experience. And for many, this makes all the difference.

Holistic Health: Integrating Body, Mind, and Spirit

At the heart of natural healing is a simple yet profound principle: true health is multidimensional. It's not only about eliminating physical symptoms, but about nurturing the full human experience—body, mind, and spirit. This integrative view is a defining feature of natural therapies, and it has become increasingly relevant in a modern world where stress, isolation, and lifestyle-related illnesses are on the rise.

In conventional care, health is often divided into specialties: cardiology for the heart, psychiatry for the mind, dermatology for the skin. Each system is treated in isolation, often with different providers and protocols. But the human body doesn't work in compartments, it functions as an interconnected whole. When stress affects the mind, it can also elevate blood pressure, suppress digestion, and disrupt sleep. When emotional trauma lingers, it can manifest physically as fatigue, inflammation, or immune vulnerability.

Natural health systems have long recognized this connection. Traditional Chinese Medicine (TCM), Ayurveda, and many indigenous healing systems do not separate emotional or spiritual imbalance from physical symptoms, they view them as part of the same ecosystem. Even modern science is now affirming this perspective. According to the American Psychological Association, chronic stress is linked to the six leading causes of death in the United States, including heart disease, cancer, and stroke. The CDC reports that as much as 75% of doctor visits involve complaints related to stress.

Natural therapies offer a wider range of tools to address these deeper causes. Practices like meditation, yoga, grounding (Earthing), breathwork, and nature immersion are increasingly used to support mental and emotional balance. These methods don't just manage stress symptoms; they work to shift the body's physiological state from chronic tension (sympathetic dominance) into calm and restorative mode (parasympathetic activation). This shift is critical, as it allows the body to redirect energy toward digestion, repair, immune support, and mental clarity.

Scientific research supports the value of these practices. A 2014 meta-analysis published in *JAMA Internal Medicine* found that mindfulness meditation can significantly reduce symptoms of anxiety, depression, and pain. Other studies have shown that regular grounding, whether through barefoot contact with the Earth or grounding mats, may influence cortisol rhythms, sleep quality, and markers of inflammation, though more research is needed. These are not fringe ideas, they are increasingly supported by evidence and used in integrative clinics and hospital wellness programs around the world.

The spiritual dimension of health, often overlooked in conventional models, is another important layer of holistic care. This doesn't necessarily refer to religion, it refers to connection, purpose, and inner alignment. Whether through prayer, nature connection, energy healing, or simply moments of stillness and reflection, many people report that tending to their spiritual well-being enhances their resilience, improves mood, and gives meaning to their healing journey.

Studies have begun to explore this connection as well and found that people with strong spiritual or religious practices reported better coping skills, lower levels of depression, and greater satisfaction with life, especially when managing chronic illness. Another study from Harvard School of Public Health concluded that spiritual well-being was associated with lower rates of burnout and better overall health among healthcare workers.

Holistic health doesn't promise perfection. But it does offer a different path, one that invites individuals to care for themselves not just as bodies with symptoms, but as whole beings with stories, emotions, values, and a desire for meaning. This approach doesn't reject conventional medicine; it expands the vision of what healthcare can be.

In a fragmented world, natural therapies offer a unifying framework. They help restore what often gets lost in modern medicine: the human experience at the center of care.

Supporting Long-Term Health

One of the most important pillars of natural health is its strong emphasis on preventive care. Rather than waiting for symptoms to signal that something is wrong, natural approaches aim to support balance, resilience, and vitality from the ground up, before health problems take root. In today's world, where lifestyle-related conditions are on the rise, this preventive mindset is more important than ever.

Chronic diseases have become the leading cause of death and disability worldwide. In the United States alone, the Centers for Disease Control and Prevention (CDC) reports that six in ten adults have a chronic health condition, and four in ten are living with two or more. These conditions are often linked to factors such as nutrition, physical activity, stress, sleep, and exposure to environmental stressors, all areas where natural health strategies can offer meaningful support.

Natural prevention begins with everyday habits. Whole-food nutrition, regular movement, restorative sleep, time in nature, and practices that reduce stress and restore emotional balance are all considered core components of a wellness lifestyle. Rather than addressing health only when symptoms appear, this approach builds a foundation that supports energy, mental clarity, and long-term function.

Scientific research supports the benefits of many of these practices. For example, omega-3 fatty acids, found in flaxseed, walnuts, and fish oil, have been widely studied for their role in reducing systemic inflammation, a contributing factor in many chronic conditions. A 2021 meta-analysis in *The Lancet* found that omega-3 intake was associated with improved cardiovascular outcomes and lower risk of mortality in at-risk populations.

Another preventive category receiving increased attention is adaptogenic herbs, plant-based compounds traditionally used to help the body manage stress. Herbs such as ashwagandha, rhodiola, and holy basil have been explored for their potential to support mood, energy, and hormonal balance in people facing chronic stress. While more clinical research is underway, these herbs are widely used as part of long-term wellness plans in both Eastern and Western natural medicine traditions.

Preventive care also includes movement practices like walking, tai chi, or yoga, which support musculoskeletal strength, lymphatic circulation, and cognitive health. In the realm of mental and emotional well-being, daily mindfulness, meditation, or grounding exercises help regulate the nervous system and build emotional resilience, both key factors in long-term wellness.

One of the unique strengths of these strategies is their suitability for daily life. They are not just temporary interventions or responses to symptoms, but lifelong habits that can be sustained without harsh side effects or dependency. Whether it's starting the day with a nutrient-dense breakfast, spending time outdoors, or creating space for emotional rest and reflection, preventive care becomes a way of living, not a protocol.

In this sense, natural therapies are not just health solutions, they are health practices. By integrating these tools into daily life, individuals can reduce their long-term risk of imbalance and build the internal conditions for wellness to thrive. Prevention becomes personal, empowering, and rooted in choice, offering a steady path toward health that honors the whole person, every day.

Environmental and Ethical Considerations

Natural therapies offer more than personal wellness; they reflect a broader commitment to environmental sustainability and ethical responsibility. For many people, choosing herbal remedies, organic foods, or nature-based practices is not just about physical health. It's also about supporting ecosystems, respecting traditional knowledge, and participating in a more conscious way of living.

The connection between health and environmental impact is becoming increasingly visible. Industrial food systems and pharmaceutical manufacturing both contribute to pollution, resource depletion, and biodiversity loss. According to the United Nations Food and Agriculture Organization (FAO), agriculture accounts for nearly one-quarter of global greenhouse gas emissions, with industrial farming practices contributing significantly through chemical fertilizers, soil degradation, and deforestation.

In contrast, many natural products are produced through sustainable farming and harvesting methods. Organic farming, for instance, avoids synthetic pesticides and fertilizers, which helps protect pollinators, preserve soil quality, and reduce water contamination. Choosing organic or biodynamic foods and herbs not only reduces your exposure to chemical residues, but it also supports farming systems that work with nature rather than against it.

The herbal supplement industry, once unregulated and prone to overharvesting, has seen a growing shift toward responsible sourcing standards. Organizations like the American Herbal Products Association (AHPA) and initiatives like FairWild have established guidelines to ensure that medicinal plants are harvested ethically and sustainably. This includes protecting endangered species, supporting indigenous harvesting traditions, and ensuring fair compensation for workers in the global botanical supply chain.

For example, herbs like Rhodiola rosea and Goldenseal, both in high demand for their adaptogenic and antimicrobial properties, have been subject to overharvesting in the wild. But increased consumer awareness has led to more regulated cultivation efforts and certifications that protect native populations while still allowing access to their benefits.

In this way, choosing natural therapies becomes a form of advocacy, supporting supply chains that prioritize ecological balance and social fairness. When you choose a sustainably sourced herbal tea or an organic supplement, you are not just investing in your own health. You are also supporting farming communities, protecting medicinal biodiversity, and helping to preserve traditional ecological knowledge that has guided plant medicine for generations.

Even beyond products, many natural therapies are inherently low-impact and non-invasive. Practices such as meditation, tai chi, breathwork, or grounding require no packaging, no manufacturing, and no physical waste. They promote health by fostering inner awareness, nervous system regulation, and emotional balance, without consuming natural resources or contributing to pollution.

This minimalist footprint stands in quiet contrast to the carbon-intensive production and disposal of medical plastics, pharmaceuticals, and high-tech diagnostic tools. While these tools are essential in many situations, it is equally valuable to support options that maintain health without drawing heavily from the planet's resources.

As consumers become more informed and value-driven, many are asking deeper questions about their health choices: Where was this product made? How were the workers treated? What is its environmental cost? Natural health offers an opportunity to align personal wellness with planetary well-being, creating a synergy between self-care and sustainability.

In a time of ecological uncertainty and rising chronic illness, this alignment is not only refreshing, but also vital. Healing, in the truest sense, extends beyond the individual. It includes the communities we live in, the land we depend on, and the values we carry forward. Natural therapies allow us to live in greater integrity with all of these.

The Future of Natural Therapies

As we look ahead, natural therapies are poised to play an increasingly meaningful role in the evolution of healthcare. No longer seen as alternative or fringe, many of these approaches are being embraced as part of a broader movement toward personalized, preventive, and integrative care. From ancient herbal traditions to cutting-edge nutrition science, natural therapies are beginning to align more closely with modern tools such as genomics, microbiome analysis, wearable health tracking, and lifestyle-based medicine.

The global healthcare landscape is changing. Chronic conditions, mental health challenges, and environmental stressors continue to place pressure on traditional healthcare systems. In response, more individuals and practitioners are turning to strategies that focus on the whole person, rather than isolated symptoms. Natural therapies are increasingly part of that conversation, not as replacements for conventional medicine, but as powerful complements that fill in the gaps where lifestyle, nutrition, and daily habits play a central role.

At the same time, growing investment in research is helping to validate many of these ancient practices through a modern lens. Clinical trials on botanical compounds, nutritional interventions, mind-body techniques, and environmental health tools are expanding rapidly. Government bodies like the National Center for Complementary and Integrative Health (NCCIH) are funding studies that explore how natural approaches can support resilience, recovery, and quality of life.

Technology is also playing a role. Digital health platforms now make it easier to track nutrient intake, monitor stress responses, and personalize supplement protocols based on individual data. These innovations are helping to bridge the gap between tradition and innovation, making natural therapies more accessible, measurable, and relevant to the needs of modern life.

But beyond science and systems, the future of natural health is deeply human. People are searching for more than just treatment, they are seeking meaning, empowerment, and sustainable ways to feel well in body, mind, and spirit. Natural therapies provide tools to support that journey, not only by addressing discomfort, but by encouraging greater awareness of how we live, what we consume, how we connect, and what truly matters.

As the challenges of modern living continue to evolve, be it stress, burnout, chronic inflammation, or environmental disruption, so too does the need for health strategies that are proactive, adaptable, and grounded in nature. Natural therapies offer that foundation. They invite individuals to take an active role in their wellness, to reconnect with their bodies, and to make small daily choices that build lasting vitality over time.

In this way, the relevance of natural therapies will not diminish, but will grow. Whether integrated into conventional care plans or practiced independently as part of daily life, these approaches represent not just a trend, but a return to principles that are both timeless and urgently needed.

Natural health is not the future of medicine alone. It is the future of how we care for ourselves, our communities, and our planet. And it starts with a simple shift: to live more in balance, more consciously, and more in tune with the healing potential that already exists within and around us.

Simple and Trusted Natural Health Approaches

In a world that often feels chaotic, overbooked, and overstimulated, many people believe that living a naturally healthy lifestyle requires dramatic changes, major diet overhauls, daily routines packed with rituals, or an abundance of free time that most people simply don't have. This perception can be especially discouraging for those already navigating ongoing wellness challenges, exhaustion, or demanding work schedules.

That's why *The Medicine-Free, Illness-Free Series* was created: to show that natural health can be simple, accessible, and trusted, even for the busiest lives. You don't need to spend hours in the kitchen, attend weekly wellness retreats, or eliminate everything you enjoy. Instead, you can begin with small, sustainable shifts, just like taking a daily supplement or adding one supportive practice at a time.

This series focuses on science-informed strategies that are as easy to integrate as conventional routines and are designed to work in harmony with the body's natural rhythms. Each approach is grounded not only in research, but also in real-world user feedback, highlighting what people actually find helpful and sustainable in their daily lives. Whether you're starting with a medicinal mushroom capsule, a grounding mat under your desk, or a daily herbal tonic, these practices offer practical, low-effort options that many people use to support energy, digestion, mood, focus, immune balance, and more.

The solutions introduced in the series, ranging from whole-food-based herbal supplements and amino acids to medicinal mushrooms, animal organ supplements, and mineral-rich protocols, are designed for real-world lifestyles. They're well-suited for those who aren't looking to overhaul everything at once but still want to explore ways to support their well-being and clarity of mind.

These methods are inspired by timeless traditions and informed by modern research, and they offer a thoughtful complement to conventional care for those seeking a more natural approach. While natural therapies do not replace essential medical treatment, they may offer additional support for maintaining balance and vitality in everyday life.

Most importantly, these approaches are approachable. You won't need to eliminate all your favorite foods, start meditating for an hour each morning, or buy an expensive blender. Instead, you'll find that well-being can feel more manageable when the tools you use are rooted in nature and designed to align with your body's needs.

The Medicine-Free, Illness-Free Series is your guide to doing just that. Whether you're experiencing occasional fatigue, digestive discomfort, or stress, or simply want to feel more balanced in your daily life, this series offers a clear and achievable path to explore natural wellness options that fit you.

This is not about perfection. It's about practical support for real people who want to feel more energized, live with greater ease, and gradually discover what helps them thrive. One step at a time.

The Medicine-Free, Illness-Free Series

Welcome to *The Medicine-Free, Illness-Free Series*, a comprehensive, nature-based roadmap designed to support your health and vitality through simple, sustainable practices. This series was created for real people with real lives: busy professionals, caregivers, those navigating ongoing health challenges, and anyone seeking more energy, balance, and clarity, without complicated routines or unwanted side effects.

As introduced in earlier chapters, many people today face persistent issues like fatigue, poor sleep, stress, digestive discomfort, and mental fog. The good news? Many have found meaningful support through natural strategies that are easy to integrate into daily life. These aren't extreme programs or major lifestyle overhauls, they're science-informed, real-world practices that meet you where you are and grow with you over time.

In the previous chapter, we explored why natural health is more relevant than ever. More than a philosophy, it's a practical, root-cause approach built on whole-food nutrition, gentle daily rhythms, and the wisdom of nature. These strategies don't fight your body; they work with it. Whether your goals are better focus, emotional stability, digestive comfort, or overall resilience, natural health offers tools that empower, not overwhelm.

What This Series Offers

The Medicine-Free, Illness-Free Series is your go-to resource for practical, research-informed natural strategies that are easy to apply. Each volume focuses on a single modality or system—herbs, mushrooms, organ supplements, amino acids, grounding, detox, and more—offering clear guidance to help you choose what works best for you.

Together, the 10 books provide a comprehensive yet flexible wellness framework that supports both daily health maintenance and targeted support. Here's a brief overview of what you'll find in each book:

The Medicine-Free, Illness-Free Series: Why Natural Health Is the Future

Explore why millions of people are turning to nature-aligned strategies to support their wellness. This foundational volume introduces the core science and philosophy behind natural approaches to health, and how they may support your sense of balance, vitality, and overall well-being.

The Medicine-Free, Illness-Free Series: Herbal Therapy

Learn how the world's most time-tested plants may support digestion, energy, relaxation, immune strength, and more. Discover practical ways to include them in your routine and how to choose herbs that match your personal needs and constitution.

The Medicine-Free, Illness-Free Series: Mushroom Therapy

Discover the unique compounds found in medicinal mushrooms that may support immunity, cognitive function, and stress resilience. This book explains how to use mushrooms such as Reishi, Lion's Mane, and Cordyceps in a daily supplement.

The Medicine-Free, Illness-Free Series: Animal Organ Therapy

Explore how nutrient-dense organ supplements, like liver, heart, and kidney, may provide highly bioavailable vitamins, minerals, and peptides. Learn how these traditional foods may support foundational wellness in areas like energy, endurance, and metabolic balance.

The Medicine-Free, Illness-Free Series: Amino Acid Therapy

Uncover the role of amino acids, the building blocks of life, in supporting mood, focus, muscle strength, and nervous system health. This volume shows how targeted amino acid support may help restore clarity, resilience, and emotional well-being.

The Medicine-Free, Illness-Free Series: HOPED Protocol

Learn the five foundational nutrient categories—High Fiber, Omega-3s & Antioxidants, Probiotics, Enzymes, and Vitamin D—and how to implement them as a core wellness strategy. HOPED is simple, actionable, and designed for everyday consistency.

The Medicine-Free, Illness-Free Series: Detoxification Therapy

Discover a gentle, nature-based approach to support your body's natural detoxification processes, promote balance, and encourage overall vitality using simple, practical techniques.

The Medicine-Free, Illness-Free Series: Grounding Therapy

Explore the science and practice of grounding (earthing), the natural process of reconnecting with the Earth's electrical field. Learn how this subtle practice may help support nervous system regulation, sleep quality, and emotional balance.

The Medicine-Free, Illness-Free Series: Diet, Lifestyle and Emotional Well-being

While drastic changes are not required, this volume introduces simple habits that promote long-term balance, covering food, movement, sleep, and emotional self-regulation in a way that aligns with the rest of your natural health plan.

The Medicine-Free, Illness-Free Series: Integrative Therapies for Everyday Health

This final volume brings together insights from the entire series, offering user-reported tools to help support everyday wellness goals, such as energy, digestion, sleep, immunity, and emotional resilience. It serves as a cross-reference for applying the therapies in complementary ways, helping you navigate your health journey with clarity and confidence.

A Science-Backed, Real-World Tested Method

In *The Medicine-Free, Illness-Free Series*, we introduce a unique, structured method for exploring natural supplements, one that blends scientific insight with real-world observations. Rather than relying solely on clinical studies or anecdotal reports, we combine both perspectives to give you a well-rounded, user-friendly understanding of each natural solution.

This balanced approach helps answer the most important questions: What does science suggest about this supplement's potential? What are people actually experiencing when they use it? Which health goals do people turn to it for most often?

Our method reflects a commitment to transparency, education, and practicality, so you can explore these natural options with clarity and confidence.

Our Four-Part Analysis Method

1. Science-Informed Solution Benefits

We begin by reviewing peer-reviewed studies, traditional usage patterns, and emerging scientific literature to understand the possible mechanisms and effects of each supplement. This provides a foundation of what is known, hypothesized, or being actively researched, offering a science-informed perspective to guide your exploration.

2. Customer-Reported Solution Benefits

We analyze large sets of customer reviews from publicly available platforms to understand how these supplements are being used in daily life. This includes what benefits people say they notice most often and how they describe their experiences.

Our focus is on patterns of what users commonly report, rather than isolated stories. This real-world layer helps connect the theory to practical, everyday outcomes.

3. Use Case Patterns & Feedback Insights

Within the customer-reported section, we highlight:

Use Case Patterns Observed – What kinds of goals or wellness concerns people most commonly use each supplement for.

Feedback Insights – How users describe the impact in their own words, including sentiment, language tone, and satisfaction cues.

Most Reported Benefits – A percentage-based summary showing which benefits are mentioned most often in reviews.

This structured summary lets you see what real people are using the supplement for, and how frequently those benefits are reported.

4. No Brand Promotion—Just Trusted Guidance

This series does not promote specific products or brands. Instead, we offer education and a decision-making framework. For those looking for high-quality sources, recommended supplement types and vetted options are available at AshiHealing.com.

Why This Method Matters

In today's crowded supplement market, it can be hard to separate hype from helpful information. That's why we created this approach, to empower you with insights drawn from scientific research, real-world usage patterns and satisfaction trends, and clear summaries that help you compare options and set expectations

You won't find exaggerated claims or one-size-fits-all solutions here. Instead, you'll find a practical, transparent method that reflects how real people are exploring natural wellness, with science as a guide and personal experience as a reference.

Whether you're considering herbs, mushrooms, amino acids, or other supplements, this method gives you a safe and structured way to learn how others are using these tools, and how they might fit into your own wellness journey.

A Personal Commitment from Dr. Forest Yin

Every approach, strategy, and supplement featured in *The Medicine-Free, Illness-Free Series* has been personally explored. Before sharing any recommendations with clients or readers, I take the time to experience it myself, observing how it affects energy, mood, sleep, digestion, and focus.

This hands-on approach allows me to understand each therapy not just through science, or just through other people's experiences. It adds a personal layer of insight to the research and user-reported feedback that shape this series.

My goal is simple: to help you find natural, sustainable solutions that feel doable, helpful, and aligned with how lasting wellness begins, by reconnecting with your body's own rhythms and innate intelligence.

How to Use This Series

Each book in *The Medicine-Free, Illness-Free Series* is designed to stand alone, offering in-depth, practical guidance on a specific category of natural therapies. Together, they form a cohesive wellness system that helps you explore a range of nature-based strategies to support your health in sustainable, manageable ways.

You can start anywhere. While many readers begin with *Why Natural Health Is the Future* to understand the foundational ideas, such as the importance of root-cause thinking and the benefits of gentle, nature-aligned care, each book builds on the last, allowing you to deepen your understanding and apply new tools at your own pace.

Start Where You Need: Choose the volume that most closely aligns with your current wellness priorities or personal curiosity. Whether it's herbal therapy, amino acids, grounding, or detoxification support, each book offers actionable insights you can implement right away. And while every volume stands on its own, the full series is designed to work synergistically, helping you build a personalized, whole-body wellness routine over time.

Build Your Routine: The strategies offered in this series are meant to be simple, flexible, and easy to integrate. Whether you're looking to support your energy, digestion, focus, or overall vitality, you'll find options that fit into everyday life without requiring dramatic changes or complex regimens.

Use as a Reference: The tenth book, *Integrative Therapies for Everyday Health*, serves as a helpful cross-reference for daily wellness concerns. It offers science-informed guidance on how the therapies featured across the series may be used in complementary ways to support overall well-being and resilience in a variety of everyday situations.

A Journey Toward Your Well-being

The Medicine-Free, Illness-Free Series is your invitation to explore nature-based solutions that support real change, physically, mentally, and emotionally. While some people may notice benefits in the first few days or weeks, the deeper strength of these practices lies in their cumulative impact over time. The more consistently you support your body with natural, science-informed tools, the more you may notice balance, energy, and resilience unfolding naturally.

By embracing this lifestyle, you're choosing a proactive path, one rooted in simplicity, sustainability, and whole-person care. These therapies are not quick fixes or miracles, they are gentle and practical methods that can support your body's ability to adapt, balance, and thrive.

Thank you for joining us on this journey. As you explore each book in the series, keep in mind that transformation doesn't always begin with a prescription. Sometimes, it begins with a deeper connection to the rhythms of nature, a shift in perspective, and the willingness to take one small step at a time.

This book is part of a larger journey toward sustainable wellness. To explore more natural health strategies or receive personalized guidance, visit AshiHealing.com.

Welcome to a new path of effortless, natural living. Let's begin..

About The Author

Dr. Forest Yin (Jie Yin) is a licensed acupuncturist, herbalist, and Doctor of Acupuncture and Oriental Medicine (DAOM). He serves as a professor and doctoral advisor at the University of East West Medicine (UEWM) and is the founder of Ashi Healing and Acupuncture Inc. With extensive experience in Traditional Chinese Medicine (TCM) and natural health, Dr. Yin integrates a wide range of holistic therapies, forming the foundation of *The Medicine-Free, Illness-Free Series.*

Before devoting his career fully to natural healing, Dr. Yin worked in the high-tech and financial sectors with both large corporations and fast-paced startups. These experiences gave him firsthand insight into the chronic stress and burnout common in modern life. Inspired to seek sustainable strategies for long-term wellness, he turned to the wisdom of nature and the depth of Chinese medicine.

Dr. Yin's clinical experience and ongoing research have helped shape practical wellness protocols that focus on balance, energy, and lifestyle-based health support. His work emphasizes simple, science-informed approaches that align with the body's natural rhythms and support overall resilience.

Driven by a mission to empower others, he created *The Medicine-Free, Illness-Free Series* to share accessible natural strategies that fit seamlessly into busy lives. His approach blends ancient healing principles with modern insight, helping people feel more energized, focused, and in tune with their long-term health goals.

Continue Your Wellness Journey

This book is just the beginning. True wellness is a lifelong journey, and you don't have to walk it alone. The Ashi Healing ecosystem is here to support you every step of the way with personalized guidance, nature-based solutions, and a shared mission: to help more people experience the benefits of natural health.

Personalized Virtual Consultation

If you're ready for expert guidance tailored to your specific needs, you can schedule a private virtual consultation with Dr. Forest Yin at AshiHealing.com. These one-on-one sessions offer a personalized supplement and herbal plan based on your current wellness goals, lifestyle, and health history, helping you create a sustainable path forward using time-tested, natural approaches.

In-Person Consultation and Acupuncture

If you're located in the San Francisco Bay Area, Dr. Yin also provides in-person consultations and acupuncture sessions at the University of East West Medicine (UEWM) campus in Sunnyvale, California, where he also teaches in the doctoral program for Traditional Chinese Medicine. This serene, professional setting offers a welcoming space for personalized care. All visits, virtual or in-person, can be scheduled through AshiHealing.com.

Supplement Recommendation Plans

Each wellness protocol discussed in this book has a corresponding supplement plan available on Fullscript, featuring practitioner-trusted, food-based formulas. These curated plans make it easy to take action without guesswork, offering clear, guided steps for nutritional support.

You can access them directly at:

https://us.fullscript.com/welcome/ashi-healing,

or simply start from AshiHealing.com.

Explore the Complete Book Series

This book is part of *The Medicine-Free, Illness-Free Series*, a 10-book collection designed to help you support your long-term health and vitality through natural methods. Each volume introduces a unique modality—from herbs and mushrooms to detoxification, grounding, amino acids, and more—so you can build your wellness path one step at a time.

Refer to the Series Overview chapter or visit AshiHealing.com to explore the full collection.

Support the Natural Health Movement

If this book has inspired you, and you believe more people should have access to clear, trustworthy information about natural health, consider supporting our mission.

The Ashi Healing Foundation *(AshiHealing.org)* is a nonprofit organization dedicated to public education, natural health awareness, and holistic wellness outreach. Your tax-deductible donation helps expand access to these tools and empowers more individuals to explore safe, evidence-informed approaches to well-being.

To contribute, visit AshiHealing.org and join the movement for a healthier, freer world.

Connect and Stay Inspired

Your healing journey doesn't end here.

Follow **Dr. Forest Yin** for more healing stories, tips, and inspiration:

Instagram, TikTok, YouTube, and X: @DrForestYin

Facebook: @DrForestYin1

LinkedIn: linkedin.com/in/forest-yin

Ready to Take the Next Step?

Scan the QR code below to visit AshiHealing.com, your starting point for virtual consultations, supplement plans, and more resources.

Your journey toward sustainable, natural wellness begins now.

Made in the USA
Monee, IL
28 May 2025

18293467R00059